Chakras for Beginners:

A complete guide for beginners to awaken and balance chakras to radiate positive energy and for spiritual healing and mindfulness

By Gary Jay

Table of Content

Introduction 1

What are chakras? 2

How Chakras Works 7

Why You Need To Balance Your Chakras To Cope With a Modern Lifestyle 14

The Seven Chakras 17

How to identify imbalance in chakras and Techinques and Affirmation to Balance Each 37

When and where to practise chakra balance 53

Chakra Meditation: 8 Steps To Practice 54

Questions for self examination 58

Introduction

I want to thank you and congratulate you for downloading the book Chances are that you already have some awareness of the word 'chakras'. Perhaps you've seen pictures, overheard conversations, or lightly dabbled in the energy systems of the body. Many in the western world are unfamiliar with what the chakras are, and how they affect our everyday lives, including our health!

The interesting thing about chakras is that, like gravity, whether or not you are paying attention to them, they play a role in your emotional, physical, and spiritual health.

Even if you are new to exploring holistic health and alternative medicine, or even other religious ideas and theosophical pursuits, having a firm understanding of this intricate energy system will definitely benefit everyone.

What are chakras?

Chakras are simply energy centers within the body. This ancient Sanskrit word literally translates as, "wheels of light". These wheels of light are located vertically in the center of your body, aligned approximately with your spine. Each chakra influences and represents a specific region of the body. As you learn how each affects your health, you can also learn how to improve the quality of your overall state by opening, clearing, strengthening, and understanding your chakras.

The Sanskrit word Chakra literally translates to wheel or disk. In yoga, meditation, and Ayurveda, this term refers to wheels of energy throughout the body. There are seven main chakras, which align the spine, starting from the base of the spine through to the crown of the head. To visualize a chakra in the body, imagine a swirling wheel of energy where matter and consciousness meet. This invisible energy, called Prana, is vital life force, which keeps us vibrant, healthy, and alive.

The Importance of the Main Chakras in the Body

These swirling wheels of energy correspond to massive nerve centers in the body. Each of the seven main chakras contains bundles of nerves and major organs as well as our psychological, emotional, and spiritual states of being. Since everything is moving, it's essential that our seven main chakras stay open, aligned, and fluid. If there is a blockage, energy cannot flow. Think of something as simple as your bathtub drain. If you allow too much hair to go into the drain, the bathtub will back up with water, stagnate and eventually bacteria and mold will grow. So is too with our bodies and the chakras. A bathtub is simple; it's physical so the fix is easy.

Keeping a chakra open is a bit more of a challenge, but not so difficult when you have awareness. Since mind, body, soul, and spirit are intimately connected, awareness of an imbalance in one area will help bring the others back into balance. Take for example, a wife, who has recently lost her husband. She develops acute bronchitis, which remains in the chest, and then gets chest pains each time she coughs. The whole heart chakra is affected in this case. If she realizes the connection between the loss and the bronchitis, healing will occur much faster if she honors the grieving process and treats that as well as the physical ailment.

The Chakras of Matter

The first three chakras, starting at the base of the spine are chakras of matter. They are more physical in nature.

First Chakra: The Muladhara is the chakra of stability, security, and our basic needs. It encompasses the first three vertebrae, the bladder, and the colon. When this chakra is open, we feel safe and fearless.

Second Chakra: The Svadhisthana chakra is our creativity and sexual center. It is located above the pubic bone, below the navel, and is responsible for our creative expression.

Third Chakra: The Manipura chakra means lustrous gem and it's the area from the navel to the breastbone. The third chakra is our source of personal power.

The Fourth Chakra: The Connection Between Matter and Spirit

Located at the heart center, the fourth chakra, anahata is at the middle of the seven and unites the lower chakras of matter and the upper chakras of spirit. The fourth is also spiritual but serves as a bridge between our body, mind, emotions, and spirit. The heart chakra is our source of love and connection.

When we work through our physical chakras, or the first three, we can open the spiritual chakras more fully.

The Chakras of Spirit

Fifth Chakra: The Vishuddha chakra is the fifth chakra, located in the area of the throat. This is our source of verbal expression and the ability to speak our highest truth. The fifth chakra includes the neck, thyroid, and parathyroid glands, jaw, mouth, and tongue.

Sixth Chakra: The Ajna chakra is located in between the eyebrows. It is also referred to the "third eye" chakra. Ajna is our center of intuition. We all have a sense of intuition but we may not listen to it or heed its warnings. Focus on opening the sixth chakra will help you hone this ability.

Seventh Chakra: The Sahaswara chakra or the "thousand petal lotus" chakra is located at the crown of the head. This is the chakra of enlightenment and spiritual connection to our higher selves, others, and ultimately, to the divine. It is located at the crown of the head.

How Chakras Works

It's generally considered to be best to open the chakras from the lower chakras up. So you make sure that first the Root chakra is open and than you proceed to the Sacral chakra, then Navel, Heart, Throat, Third Eye and finally Crown chakra.

The Root chakra is the foundation. When the Root chakra is open, you're able to feel secure and welcome. Having opened this chakra, you'll feel you'll have territory.

Only when you feel secure and welcome, are you able to express feelings and sexuality appropriately, the domain of the Sacral chakra. This is generally contact with one person at a time. Feelings get you an idea of what you want and when you are aware of that, you can open the Navel chakra, to assert your wants, to decide upon them. This assertion is something that's done between people, in groups, in social situations. Being able to deal with social situations, you can form affectionate relationships, which is the domain of the Heart chakra.

This tames the aggression of the Navel chakra. When relationships are formed, you are able to express yourself, by the Throat chakra. This is also the basis of thinking, which makes insight possible, by opening the Third Eye chakra. When all these chakras are open, you're ready for the Crown chakra, to develop wisdom, self-awareness and awareness of the whole.

What period of time you spend on each chakra, is something you'll have to find out for yourself. Be aware of how you feel and what you do and don't do. Notice if you really do need to open certain chakras and if you can sustain higher ones. It's probably a process of years, if not decades, although you'll be enjoying benefits immediately. It will not always be necessary to rigidly follow the order of the chakras, as long as you're aware of what's happening with you.

The test for the chakras can help you determine which ones you'll need to open. It's mostly a matter of being aware what your state is. To develop this awareness, it's a good idea to do meditation. That also helps to balance the chakras, and is particularly helpful when you have overactive chakras. Vipassana and Zen meditation are in particular recommended.

How chakras affects lifestyle and well being

Around the world, people are looking for answers and better ways to improve their wellbeing that they are not finding in their daily lives. So, it is probably no surprise that ancient forms of therapy are making a comeback as they can provide a better sense of wellbeing for those who lead busy lives.

One practice that has made a strong comeback is chakras and their proper alignment in the body that better directs the flow of energy. But what are chakras and how can they be used to help people get what they need out of their lives?

The direction of energy in your body is crucial to living a better lifestyle and augmenting the feeling of wellbeing. In many cases, a person's feeling about their own health is greatly influenced by the alignment of energy in their bodies. By using traditional methods that include meditation and prayer, you can help your body regain the alignment it once had so that you feel better and become healthier.

Chakras are not the end-all, be-all when it comes to your health, but you do greatly improve your lifestyle and wellbeing when you spend a few moments engaging in techniques designed to bring out your chakras so that the energy flow is constant and on-target. In fact, one of the more interesting and easy to perform methods of unleashing the energies found inside the chakras is through the use of aromatherapy.

How Chakras and Aromatherapy can Work Together?

As part of your efforts to improve your wellbeing through the proper alignment of the chakras, essential oils have proven to be a marvelous method of assisting with the spiritual growth as well as assisting with the ailments which plague the body.

Essential oils have been around for many centuries and have proven to have positive benefits on the mind as well as the body. Today, these oils are making a strong comeback as people discover the natural benefits that they bring, particularly in conjunction with the attention paid to chakras and other elements that can help provide you with better wellbeing. In addition, many essential oils may be mixed with carrier oils such as olive or coconut oils and applied to the body where the chakras can be released.

Whether breathed in through the nose, rubbed onto the body, essential oils and chakras can work together to help bring a better state of wellbeing with the body. However, it is aromatherapy that may have the most powerful effect on the body itself when working with the chakras.

Aromatherapy is where essential oils are used the most as they are breathed in where they have a positive, powerful effect on the mind. In fact, of the five senses only smell has a direct connection to the brain which is why it is so powerful.

Balancing Chakras with Aromatherapy

To achieve the proper balance between aromatherapy and chakras starts by engaging in self improvement plan that gradually takes in both methods over time so that they become part of your lifestyle. All too often, people dive into both without knowing what to expect or worse, expecting that everything will change immediately.

Instead, the proper way to engage in chakras and aromatherapy is to start slowly with just a few minutes out of your day. Aromatherapy can consist of simply putting a few drops of essential oils in an essential oil diffuser and meditating for just a few moments as the odor of the oils is breathed in. After a few sessions over the course of a week, you'll start to really feel better as your chakras start to find better balance in your body and mind.

To engage in the proper techniques over time is how you can achieve the right balance of chakras and aromatherapy so that your wellbeing is improved as it becomes a part of your lifestyle.

When it comes to finding the right aromatherapy products, Gifts Ready To Go has what you need. Offering a complete line of aromatherapy gifts that will help improve your wellbeing, including essential oils and other self improvement aids, Gifts Ready To Go is the place where you can augment your lifestyle and also find gifts that are perfect for your friends and family.

Why You Need To Balance Your Chakras To Cope With a Modern Lifestyle

Chakra centres, which are the energy vortices from which we maintain our energy flow, are constantly changing as they interact, redressing and maintaining their dynamic balance of energy. Although each of us has a different pattern of predominant chakras which define our unique energy flow, linked to each individual and their individual lifestyle, the energy chakras also affect our minute to minute energy states, as we carry out our daily activities. During an average day we can have cause to relax, become stressed, perform physical activity or reflect on life and each demands a different supply of energy from the relevant energy centres.

Examples of chakras being identified with certain lifestyles are the 1st and 2nd chakras association with physical and practical jobs and lifestyles, whereas the brow chakra is linked to creative tasks and solar plexus to an organisational activity.

Our modern changing lifestyles and multi-tasking means that our chakra balance is even more important than ever and maintaining complex relationships at work and socially requires a healthy heart chakra balance, however we can also be thrown into a situation where there is no such contact, or where our interpersonal skills are not valued, thus we have to quickly redress our chakra energies in different ways. Balancing our chakra centres in this way will help a great deal towards maintaining our physical and mental well being.

Although there is no problem when a particular chakra has dominance, the imbalance can cause other chakras to attempt to cover the roles of those being under-used and we will feel 'out of sorts' due to our energies being serviced by inappropriate energy centres. When this happens we feel lacklustre and needing a recharge.

Because the chakras are working so dynamically as we perform our daily tasks, it is important to balance them regularly so that they are optimised for our energy system. Because we are all unique there is no formula for how to balance our particular chakras, but you can use a disciplined approach using crystals associated with each energy centre.

Crystals help to amplify the energy associated with the chakra and there are correspondences associated with each crystal, which enables them to work better with a certain chakra. By knowing the correct crystals to use, chakra energy balancing can be optimised so that you always feel energized and motivated.

There are modern methods of charging crystals with certain frequencies for a desired effect, crystals charged in this way will have an amplified effect on the relevant chakra resulting in a stronger, more positive energy balance. These are known as isochronic crystals and are fast becoming the modern way to approach crystal energy work.

The Seven Chakras

The human body contains 114 chakras or energy centres, this article will only focus on the 7 primary chakras as depicted in yoga practises. The 7 primary chakras are vertically spaced along the spinal cord from the tail bone (root) up to the top of the head (crown). In a physical sense, these energy centres are a mass of nerves that govern our physical organs and our emotional or mental attributes. These wheels of light are located vertically in the center of your body, aligned approximately with your spine.

Each chakra influences and represents a specific region of the body. As you learn how each affects your health, you can also learn how to improve the quality of your overall state by opening, clearing, strengthening, and understanding your chakras.

The Seven Chakras include

1. Root Chakra
2. Sacral Chakra
3. Solar Plexus Chakra
4. Heart Chakra
5. Throat Chakra
6. Third Eye Chakra
7. Crown Chakra

The Physical Chakras

The first 3 Chakras relate to our physical attributes and base instincts. Let's take a closer look at them in order:

Root Chakra or Muladhara

The Root Chakra is the first of 7 main energy centres located at the base of your spine, it encompasses the first 3 vertebrae and is the root of your being; it has deep connections with your physical body, your environment and Mother Earth. The Root Chakra spins at the slowest rate of all the major Chakras. It relates to your physical body such as bones/teeth, Adrenal Gland, Legs, Feet and Large Intestine.

This chakra is at the root of our base instincts such as survival, security and stability. When this chakra is lacking or unbalanced; we may feel insecure, suffer from anxiety or panic attacks, and develop bowel disorders, eating disorders, bone/teeth disorders, frequently cold feet and sore legs.

When this chakra is functioning correctly, we feel safe, fearless and have good physical health in regard to the above symptoms. The colour associated with this chakra is dark red or brown and the element is earth.

Imagine you are viewing your spine as if it is an electrical cord plugging you into the base of your body. The outlet is located in the perineum region of the body, at the base of the spine. This is where the Root Chakra is located.

The root chakra represents your connection to the earth, your survival instincts, and correlates to the base of Maslow's Hierarchy of Needs.

Sacral Chakra or Svadhisthana

The second chakra is where your emotions, creativity and sexuality flows from. The Sacral Chakra is located between the navel and pelvic area. This important energy centre is responsible for regulating the health of your kidneys, pancreas, liver, adrenal glands, spleen, bladder and sexual organs.

Imbalances or blockages here can manifest the following physical and emotional issues:

* Sexual addictions
* Addiction to stimulation
* Mood swings
* Emotional over sensitivity
* Emotional dependency/instability
* Lack of desire, passion, or excitement
* Lack of sexual appetite, desire
* Poor social skills and relationship problems.

An open and healthy sacral chakra allows us to access our creative forces easily, express our emotions and our sexuality in a balanced natural way. The colour associated with this chakras vibration is orange, and the element is water.

The Sacral Chakra is also known as the sexual chakra as it corresponds directly to the reproductive organs. It also symbolizes creativity.

The Solar Plexus Chakra or Manipura

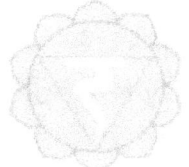

The third chakra is located between the navel and the solar plexus. This important energy centre is the seat of our ego and as such our personality. Our self-esteem, willpower and confidence flows from this chakra. It's element is fire - hence the saying "she has fire in her belly". The main challenge for this chakra is learning to use our personal power in a balanced reliable way.

Blockages or deficient energy at this chakra level may manifest the following conditions:

* Emotional outbursts
* React negatively to life circumstances
* Passive \ inactive
* Often stressed out
* Low self-esteem
* Low energy

* Weak will \ easily lead, controlled & manipulated
* Lack of confidence
* Cold, emotionally &/or physically
* Victim mentality
* Bullied &/or physical abusive

Excessive energy at this level manifests the following:

* Manipulative
* Power hungry, dominating & controlling
* Deceitful
* Overly aggressive
* Addiction to sedatives
* Hyperactive
* Need to be right \ have last word
* Overly competitive
* Arrogant
* Temper tantrums

Physical disorders:

* Eating disorders
* Diabetes
* Muscle spasms

* Hypoglycaemia
* Chronic fatigue
* Muscular disorders
* Hypertension
* Digestive disorders
* Pancreas, adrenal gall, liver & bladder disorders

You may have recognized a sick feeling in the pit of your stomach, or gotten butterflies due to anticipation. These are physical sensations associated with the activity of your solar plexus chakra! This chakra is where you would deal with issues of personal will, identity, and emotion.

Keeping this centre balanced is essential for good physical and emotional health.

The Fourth Chakra

The fourth chakra, known as the heart chakra or anahata is where physical matter meets spiritual energy. This chakra simultaneously operates on both dimensions and is considered the bridge to the upper chakras which all operate at higher frequencies on the dimension of spirit or mind. The Heart chakra is located between the chest, in the center of the breastbone; at the back its location is the first thoracic vertebra between and below the shoulder blades.

This important chakra resonates with the colour green and relates to feelings of love, self love, intimacy, relationships, forgiveness or lack of, attachments to people and devotion. This chakra corresponds with the following physical glands; Thymus, Heart, lungs, arms, hands, immune system and Circulation.

Blockages or deficiencies at this level can manifest the following emotional conditions:

* Lack of self love
* lack of empathy
* intimacy issues/sexual abuse
* antisocial/withdrawn
* intolerance of self and others
* depression
* fear of commitment/relationships
* judgemental/critical
* Excessive energy at this centre can manifest the following:

Demanding, co-dependent, clingy, jealousy, fear of abandonment.

Physical Malfunctions:

Disorders of the heart, lungs, thymus, breasts, arms, Shortness of breath, Sunken chest, Circulation problems, Asthma, Immune system deficiency, Tension between shoulder blades, pain in chest.

Balanced Characteristics include:

* Compassionate
* Loving
* Empathetic
* Self loving
* Altruistic
* Peaceful
* Balanced
* Strong immune system

The Spiritual Chakras

The top 3 chakras vibrate at much higher frequencies than the lower three. These powerful chakras that are said to operate in the realm of spirit; govern our mind, intuition, intelligence and connection to the divine.

The Throat Chakra or Vishuddha

The 5th chakra is located between the shoulders and the ears. This chakra spins at a much faster rate than the previous 4 and corresponds to our verbal expression, speaking your truth, articulating your thoughts/emotions accurately, and the physical aspects of the shoulders, thyroid gland, parathyroid glands, throat/neck, tonsils, tongue, gums, mouth and ears.

This chakra resonates with the colour sky blue and deficencies or blockages may lead to the following symptoms:

* Lies mixed messages
* Verbal abuse and shouting
* Excessive criticism (blocks the creativity)
* Secretive behaviour
* Alcoholic or drug dependencies
* Shyness \ Introversion

* Fear of speaking out
* Softly spoken
* Difficulty putting feelings into words
* Poor rhythm
* Tone deaf

Excessive energy Symptoms:

* Over talkative
* Inability to listen
* Repetitive verbal expression
* Gossiping
* Over Loud or Dominant voice
* Interrupting others

Physical Symptoms

* Stiff shoulders\neck
* Shoulder issues
* Tonsillitis
* Frequent sore throats
* Gum infections
* Frequent\chronic Bad breath
* Ear infections and other disorders
* Voice chords
* Jaw ache or locking

Communication is key for this chakra, including the expression of talents, truth, and anger. Often when we swallow our emotions, and refuse to speak up, we will find ourselves with a physical manifestation of throat issues.

Brow Chakra, Third Eye or Ajna chakra

The 6th chakra is located between the brow at the center of the head; this chakra encompasses the eyes, the pineal gland and the base of the skull. The third eye is associated with our intuition, vision, memory, imagination/visulisation, dreams, healthy sleep cycles and according to mystics - psychic abilities.

This chakra resonates a deep indigo blue or purple. Blockages or deficiencies at this chakra can produce the following symptoms:

* Poor vision\memory
* Insensitivity
* Lack of imagination
* Denial
* Lack of foresight
* Unable to remember dreams
* Unable to visualise clearly
* Frequent headaches

Excessive energy at this center can manifest the following symptoms:

* Hallucinations
* Obessive behaviour
* Delusions
* Day dreaming constantly
* Difficulty concentrating
* Nightmares
* Frequent Migraines
* Insominia
* Mental Health issues

Communication is key for this chakra, including the expression of talents, truth, and anger. Often when we swallow our emotions, and refuse to speak up, we will find ourselves with a physical manifestation of throat issues.

The Crown Chakra or Sahaswara chakra

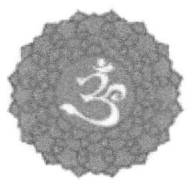

The Sahaswara chakra which translates as thousand petal lotus flower is located in the crown at the top of the skull. This chakra is associated with knowledge, enlightenment, awarness, intelligence, wisdom, our connection to others and spirituality or the divine spirit.

This chakra resonates the colours indigo to pure white. Deficiencies or blockages at this chakra can manifest the following symptoms:

* Secretive Behaviour
* Misinformation
* Lies
* Blind Faith
* Narrow mindedness
* Learning difficulties
* Greed & Materialism

* Domination of others

Over abundant energy at this chakra level manifests the following symptoms:

* Over developed intellect
* Spiritual addiction
* Dissociative behaviour
* Difficulty socialising
* Confusion
* Dissociation from body

This is your Crown Chakra and represents your connection to Divinity. It doesn't matter what religious background you come from, the crown chakra still acts as a gateway for that divine energy and connection to enter your body.

That sums up the 7 major chakras and the potential issues that deficient or excessive energy can cause. Yogi healers believe that when one is physically ill or falls under the influence of a disease/sickness it is directly related to these chakras malfunctioning. The issues tend to begin from the mind and gradually manifest into physical ailments the longer the underlying issues are left untreated.

How to identify imbalance in chakras and Techinques and Affirmation to Balance Each

There are 7 main energy centers in the body, known as chakras. Each chakra is located throughout our body so that it correlates to specific body ailment and physical dysfunctions; each energy center also houses our mental and emotional strengths. When we have a physical issue, it creates weaknesses in our emotional behavior. When we release the stale energy from the body, it can undo any tightness, stiffness, or malfunction of that area.

The clearing of the energy can also balance our emotional state of mind.

Mind-Body Balance is a two-way street: if there are certain fears and emotions we are holding on to, we experience physical restrictions, too.

If you have achiness or stiffness, or certain reoccurring emotions and fears, read along and you may find out which chakra is affected or blocked.

1st or Root Chakra

Sits at the base of your spine, at your tailbone.

Physical imbalances in the root chakra include problems in the legs, feet, rectum, tailbone, immune system, male reproductive parts and prostrate gland. Those with imbalances here are also likely to experience issues of degenerative arthritis, knee pain, sciatica, eating disorders, and constipation.

Emotional imbalances include feelings affecting our basic survival needs: money, shelter and food; ability to provide for life's necessities.

First chakra imbalances:

-you don't feel safe
-mistrust in the process of life and of others.
-disconnection with the earth and nature
-worried about basic needs
-instability
-physically: pain in lower back, elimination problems, ailments in legs or feet.

What to do....

The very best thing to do to strengthen the root chakra is to GET OUTSIDE. Go for a walk, plant something, weed or work in the garden, stand in the grass in bare feet, sit on the ground, go for a picnic, in a field, by the ocean, in a forest....

Just reconnect with the earth, you'll be amazed. I also love yoga poses for grounding. And colour therapy - RED. Protein is also important for this chakra so be sure to get enough. Find what works for you and stay with it for a week or so, things will shift.

When this chakra is balanced, we have an ability to take risks, we are creative, we are committed. We are passionate, sexual and outgoing.

When this chakra is balance, you feel supported, a sense of connection and safety to the physical world, and grounded.

The lesson of this chakra is self-preservation; we have a right to be here.

Affirmation: "I am a divine being of light, and I am peaceful, protected and secure"

2nd or Sacral Chakra

Located two inches below your navel.

Physical imbalances include sexual and reproductive issues, urinary problems, kidney dysfunctions, hip, pelvic and low back pain.

Emotional imbalances include our commitment to relationships. Our ability to express our emotions. Our ability to have fun, play based on desires, creativity, pleasure, sexuality. Fears of impotence, betrayal, addictions.

-lack of creativity

-trouble expressing desire or sensuality

-anger or jealousy

-trouble enjoying yourself or experiencing pleasure easily

-physically: fertility or sexual problems, kidney or bladder issues

What to do....

Find ways to make connection with your CREATIVITY. Choose one activity that you feel you can be creative doing. Music, dancing, singing, art, sewing, knitting, cooking, building something, writing, collaborating with someone can be fun too. Maybe brainstorm an idea together and really let yourself get lost in the creative process. Orange foods will support you too.

The lesson of this chakra is to honor others.

Affirmation: "I am radiant, beautiful and strong and enjoy a healthy and passionate life"

3rd or Solar Plexus Chakra

Located three inches above your navel.

Physical imbalances include digestive problems, liver dysfunction, chronic fatigue, high blood pressure, diabetes, stomach ulcers, pancreas and gallbladder issues, colon diseases.

Emotional imbalances include issues of personal power and self-esteem, our inner critic comes out. Fears of rejection, criticism, physical appearances.

Third chakra imbalances:

-lack of self confidence or decision making

-no sense of purpose

-depression

-aggression or arrogance

-physically: slow metabolism, weight gain, poor digestion.

What to do....

LAUGH!!! This chakra is mobilized by laughter, truly the best medicine (my Nana....right again) Funny movies, hang out with funny people. My personal fave that is guaranteed to pull me out of any funk is funny cat videos. They're so ridiculous.

Engage your core muscles with some exercise. Try surrounding yourself with yellow, it's not a color we normally choose for decor but it always feels good! Daffodils, yellow blanket, towels or pillows. I'm a big fan of colored glass, I usually pick it up at the thrift store and it's on pretty much every window ledge in the house. I think if I feel better at home I'm more likely to radiate that into the world when I'm interacting with others.

When this chakra is balanced, we feel self-respect and self-compassion. We feel in control, assertive, confident.

The lesson of this chakra is self-acceptance.

Affirmation: "I am positively empowered and successful in all my ventures".

4th or Heart Chakra

Located at the heart.

Physical imbalances include asthma, heart disease, lung disease, issues with breasts, lymphatic systems, upper back and shoulder problems, arm and wrist pain.

Emotional imbalances include issues of the heart; over-loving to the point of suffocation, jealousy, abandonment, anger, bitterness. Fear of loneliness.

Fourth chakra imbalances:

-lack of compassion for self or others

-feeling like there is not enough LOVE in your life

-co-dependancy

-selfishness or intolerance

-heart, circulatory or skin problems

What to do....

I know you know.... LOVE YOURSELF sister. That's where it starts. Is there some way you could be more loving with yourself? Treating your body a little kinder by resting more, eating healthier and exercising? This WILL radiate outward to your relationships.

The more you love yourself, the more lovable you are.

When this chakra is balanced we feel joy, gratitude, love and compassion, forgiveness flows freely, trust is gained.

The lesson of this chakra is I Love.

Affirmation: "Love is the answer to everything in life, and I give and receive love effortlessly and unconditionally"

5th or Throat Chakra

Located at the throat.

Physical imbalances include thyroid issues, sore throats, laryngitis, TMJ, ear infections, ulcers, any facial problems (chin, cheek, lips, tongue problems) neck and shoulder pain.

Emotional imbalances include issues of self-expression through communication, both spoken or written. Fear of no power or choice. No willpower or being out of control.

Fifth chakra imbalances:

-trouble expressing or communicating

-weak voice

-lying (even white ones are no good)

-talking too much (not listening)

-physically: sore throat, neck or shoulders. Ear trouble, thyroid imbalance.

What to do....

Be clear about what you need, SPEAK YOUR TRUTH. Speak with integrity and you have no need to worry about what others think. The right people will stay, the others will go. I love singing as a way to keep this chakra healthy. A good cup of peppermint tea and a lapis necklace never hurt either ;) Explore the site for more ways to support this chakra...

When this chakra is balanced, we have free flowing of words, expression, communication. We are honest and truthful yet firm. We are good listeners.

The lesson of this chakra is to speak up and let your voice be heard.

Affirmation: "I am tuned into the divine universal wisdom and always understand the true meaning of life situations"

6th or Third Eye Chakra

Located in the middle of the eyebrows, in the center of the forehead.

Physical imbalances include headaches, blurred vision, sinus issues, eyestrain, seizures, hearing loss, hormone function.

Emotional imbalances include issues with moodiness, volatility, and self-reflection; An inability to look at ones own fears, and to learn from others. Day-dream often and live in a world with exaggerated imagination.

Sixth chakra imbalances:

-not trusting your intuition

-feeling that imagination is unimportant

-lack of knowledge of self

-fear of success

-physically: headaches, sinus trouble, hearing problems, sleep disorders, weak concentration, overly sensitive to others emotions

What to do....

To thy known self be true....TRUST YOUR INTUITION MORE. It's ok to say "I don't feel like it". If a situation feels not quite right or if you feel a different choice should be made, then do it. You don't have to justify it. This is powerful guidance at work.

Generations past trusted this wisdom to save lives and rule empires. You'll see that when you do, there's always a reason.

When this chakra is balanced we feel clear, focused, and can determine between truth and illusion. We are open to receiving wisdom and insight.

The lesson of this chakra is to see the big picture.

Affirmation: "I am tuned into the divine universal wisdom and always understand the true meaning of life situations"

7th or Crown Chakra

Located at the top of the head.

Physical imbalance include depression, inability to learn, sensitivity to light, sound, environment.

Emotional imbalances include issues with self-knowledge and greater power.

Imbalances arise from rigid thoughts on religion and spirituality, constant confusion, carry prejudices, "analysis paralysis." Fear of alienation.

Seventh chakra imbalances:

-feeling of separateness or lonliness

-depression or escapism

-feeling lost

-lack of awareness of divine connection

-lack of joy in life

-physically: headaches, migraines, epilepsy, psychosis, high blood pressure

What to do....

Find a way to CONNECT with universal source energy, whatever that means for you. Meditation, spiritual groups, studying or spending time with a spiritual mentor. Decide what it all means for you and what you need to do to feel the most connected to it. You may find connection in simple activities too, a walk in nature perhaps.

When this chakra is balanced, we live in the present moment. We have an unshakeable trust in our inner guidance.

The lesson of this chakra is live mindfully.

After reading this, you (like me) may feel that more than one chakra is imbalanced or blocked. This is because when one is blocked, the other chakras begin to compensate and either become overactive or under-active.

Affirmation: "I am complete and one with the divine energy"

The best way to start balancing them is to start at the root chakra and work your way up to the crown chakra.

Chakra balancing affirmations can create extraordinary revolutions in our spiritual healing journey. There can be nothing more effective and transformative than using your very own power of thought to bring positive changes in your body, mind and soul.

When and where to practise chakra balance

Chakras can be practiced in the early hours of the morning or during the evening when we are off from work.

There are various places to practice Chakras. You can perform it at home or at special centers. No matter how much you read or study about it, unless you don't find time to practise doing meditation, you will not achieve the desired goals. Practising chakras balance should be in a peaceful place (or you can use Sound-cancelling headphones at other times).

Never Procrastinate. Each session is an oppurtunity to learn, cleanse and heal yourself.

Chakra Meditation: 8 Steps To Practice

The following steps describe how to practice a chakra meditation to balance and align your chakra energies. It is brought to us by Holistic Review Quarterly:

1. Chakra meditation begins by sitting in a comfortable position with your spine straight, but not ridged. You then want to focus on each part of your body starting with your feet and working up. As you do this, have that part of the body relax and let the stress melt away.

2. The next step in chakra meditation is to focus on the breath. Do not force it, but let the breathing become steady and deep. The mind will most likely wonder, just gentle bring it back to the breath and maintain the focus on each inhalation and exhalation you take. Visualize the oxygen coming into your lungs and passing into the bloodstream. Visualize it nourishing all the muscles, organs and cells of your body and then see it removing the toxins from your body which you expel with each breath.

3. Next in chakra meditation you want to visualize the beating of the heart and the perfect function of the body. See how all the parts work together in complete harmony. See how the breath sustains all these parts and the body as a whole. Become aware of how the breath is the life giving force ofthe entire organism you call your body.

4. Next in chakra meditation you should imagine a life giving energy that you are breathing in along with the air. See this energy as a yellowish orange color. See this energy encompass your entire body and infuse your aura. As this energy infuses your aura, imagine the aura growing stronger, brighter and being charged with this incredible energy. Do this step gradually, let the aura grow brighter little by little and keep this energy flowing in with each breath.

5. The next thing we want to do in chakra meditation is energize each individual chakra. Start with the root chakra in the lower back. Imagine a clockwise swirl of energy and the energy you breath in feeds this swirl and makes it strong and brighter.

We want to next imagine another source of energy that is coming up from the earth. This is the same life giving energy and it adds to the swirling energy at the root chakra.

6. Next in chakra meditation we want to move up to the sacral chakra. Then one by one the solar plex chakra, heart chakra, throat chakra, head chakra and finally the crown chakra, infusing each with the life giving energy. Take your time with this and do not worry about spending more time on one chakra if you need to. It is strongly advised to always work from the bottom, going up and not skip around. Each chakra will influence the other chakras and energizing a higher chakra before a lower chakra could have an adverse effect.

7. The last step in chakra meditation is to visualize all the chakras at once being feed by this energy coming in from the breath and up from the earth. Remember to see the chakras and your aura become brighter, clearer and super charged from this life giving energy.

8. Finally we can open our eyes and relax a couple minutes with our eyes open. Pay attention to your body and how incredible and energized you now feel. Try to practice 15 – 30 minutes each sitting. Enjoy, this is a really good, uplifting chakra meditation.

Questions for self examination

Q1. Do you often feel un-grounded and threatened in the world?
Related Chakra: Root or Base Chakra
Color: Red

Q2. Do you often feel it difficult to bond with other and/or being creative?
Related Chakra: Sacral Chakra
Color: Orange

Q3. Do you often feel like a victim and/or have a lack of direction?
Related Chakra: Solar plexus Chakra

Q4. Do you often feel jealous, fearful in relationships and hateful towards
Related Chakra: Heart Chakra
Color: Green

Q5. Do you find it hard to express yourself to others?
Related Chakra: Throat Chakra
Color: Blue

Q6. Are you mentally rigid and feel down a lot?
Related Chakra: Third eye Chakra
Color: Indigo

Q7. Do you often feel lost and lack the big picture of life?
Related Chakra: Crown Chakra
Color: Violet

Thank you again for purchasing this book!

I hope this book was able to help you to understand how the chakra system works. The next step is to implement what you've just learnt.

Finally, if you enjoyed this book, would you be kind enough to leave a review for this book on Amazon?

Thank you and good luck!

Gary Jay

www.ingramcontent.com/pod-product-compliance
Lightning Source LLC
Chambersburg PA
CBHW070358190526
45169CB00003B/1039